Healthy Eating

30 Days of Clean Eating: The Perfect Cookbook To Start A Healthy Diet And Still enjoy Some Sneaky Sweets

Table of Contents

Introduction

Congratulations on downloading your personal copy of *healthy Eating: 30 Days of Cean Eating; The Perfect Cookbook To Start A Healthy Diet And Still Enjoy Some Sneaky Sweets.* Thank you for doing so. This book has been created to make life easier for you and your busy lifestyle. After all, who has time to plan and cook a meal that takes an hour or more? These recipes are just what you have been searching for all of the time.

The following chapters will discuss some of the many of the ways you can eat healthier and at the same time keep track of the food you are consuming by using a point system.

You will discover the science of the Smart Points system since the calories set are the baseline of the value of what the food is worth. Each food added to the product will possibly raise the content of fat or sugar. Proteins are calculated into the equation to help lower the points.

The goal is to get you on the right track of choosing leaner proteins, and eating more fruits and veggies with each meal. By increasing these food items, you are lowering the unhealthy fats and consuming less sugar. You will be surprised since some of the foods are so tasty on this plan, and they don't take that long from start to finish. It's hard to believe they are 'diet' foods because, in essence, they are your healthier lifestyle looking at you!

There are plenty of books on this subject on the market; thanks again for choosing this one! Every effort was made to ensure it is full of as much useful information as possible to accommodate your way of cooking. Please enjoy!

Chapter 1: The Healthy Eating Plan

You will soon discover making a few adjustments to the way you purchase and prepare your foods is one of the key elements to a healthier and 'fitter' YOU. These are some of the secrets, so many have discovered:

Weight Loss Tips

Losing weight is never considered to be a fun event, but with the Healthy Eating plan, you can enjoy foods you never imagined you could have consumed while still on a regimen of losing weight. These are some of them to get you on the right track:

Drink Water

You cannot get more basic on any diet plan than to drink plenty of water since it has been proven to boost your metabolism between 24 to 30% over the time span of one to 1 ½ hours. One diet study discovered 44% more weight was dropped when the participant had consumed about half of a liter (approximately 17 ounces) of water about thirty minutes to an hour before mealtime.

Healthy Coconut Oil

Special fats, which are called medium chain triglycerides, are contained in the oil which is metabolized much different from other fats. Consider this; you aren't adding coconut oil to your current oil—you are replacing some of your current 'fats' which you cook with in your kitchen daily.

Eggs Count

Begin your day with eggs since they play a role in your plan of losing weight with benefits you might not have considered. Research has shown that participants who replaced a grain-based breakfast with eggs—lost more body fat and (yes) weight. Also proven was over a 36-hour period, you will consume fewer calories after eating eggs.

You don't like eggs; not a problem—you can choose a quality protein choice instead!

Coffee Please

For those of you who enjoy a morning cup of coffee—good job! Quality coffee is responsible for many health benefits and antioxidants. The caffeine can burn between 10- to 29% of fat burning as well as boosting your metabolism between 3- to 11% after having a cup of hot coffee.

Leave the high-calorie additives including sugar out of the drink which could negate the benefits including the following nutrients for your daily recommended amounts:

- Vitamin B2 (Riboflavin): 11%
- Vitamin B5 (Pantothenic Acid) 6%
- Potassium and Manganese: 3%
- B3/Niacin and Magnesium: 2%

These are the benefits from one cup daily. The tally can add up quickly if you enjoy the black liquid three or four times each day.

Tea Lovers

Choose green tea for their catechins, also called antioxidants, and are believed to work with caffeine to increase fat burning elements.

Lower the Intake of Refined Carbs

Grains and sugars are the culprits for weight gain many times because they have been stripped of their nutritious parts, including foods such as with pasta and white bread. Think about it when you indulge; your blood sugar will rapidly spike—leading to hunger, cravings, and more food intake within a few hours (via over-eating).

Lower Added Sugars

Start by leaving out sugars that are high in fructose corn syrup. These sugars are powerfully associated with the risk of type 2 diabetes, the risk of obesity, heart disease, and many other health issues. The easiest way to eliminate them is to read the labels since even 'health foods' can be consumed with sugar.

Fool Your Mindset

Consuming fewer calories will lead to a healthier weight. You can trick your mind by using a smaller plate which seems like a strange method, but the technique works. Try it the next time you prepare your dinner!

Others have discovered brushing and flossing your teeth after the evening meal is helpful. Somehow, it is a hint to your mind that you don't need that late snack; you already brushed your teeth and are prepared for bed!

Enjoy the Spices

You have heard the adage of 'variety is the spice of life.' It is sincerely true with the Weight Watchers plan; you can use spices to boost your metabolism. It has been proven that Cayenne pepper contains Capsaicin for the 'boost' effect. Enjoy them with your protein and fiber-rich foods.

Losing Weight: 80/20

As an eye-opener; you have to realize there are no 'magic' foods that will help you lose weight; you only need to consume less energy than your body needs to drop the pounds. Of course, you already realize there is nothing simple or easy when it comes to sticking with typical diet plans.

You are seeking a way to diet that will work for you individually, that will make you stick to the plan, and not leave because you have been deprived of good tasting, and yes healthier meal choices to reach your desired weight goals. You have to find a plan that will 'click' for you.

The healthy eating plan considers if you use the 80/20 rule; you can stick to the diet plan for 80% of the time and sneak away with some chocolate or other craved foods for the 20% time span. It will give you the willpower to tackle the rest of the hours using the unique recipes provided within this book.

How the Healthy Eating Points Are Calculated

Everyone has heard the commercials of how many pounds have been lost on the Weight Watcher's System. Did you ever wonder how the system works?

It happens like this. A team of experts are placed in charge by the Chief Scientific Officer to determine how many points members need to consider in relation to his/her weight, height, gender, and age.

The equation is calculated to determine the 'member's' resting metabolic rate or the number of calories your body can burn daily. Once that number is discovered, the Weight Watcher teams focus on determining how many calories should be consumed daily to lose one to two pounds each week.

That is how you derive the number of points for each of the items on the chosen menu. You have calculated your allowances using a special table which provides you with the number of points allowed daily.

For example; this is the information used from the chart for a female individual who is 63 years old, 184 pounds, and 5'1"tall. The total is 26 points.

You can also use the food calculator on the same link that uses the food counter for protein, carbs, fat, and fiber so you can see how many point values are included in a specific meal. For example, a particular recipe has 16 g of protein; 2 grams of carbs, 3 g fat, and 0 grams of fiber. The total would be 2 points for that meal according to the chart.

Test your limits with this handy chart provided by the Healthy Weight Forum. It is not the "official" Weight Watchers tool because you would have to be a member to receive that information.

Sample Menu

These are just a few examples of a typical day using menus with corresponding Smart - Points values. The information provided is so you can see how to break down the daily items of foods you consume with its corresponding points if you do not have a recipe or chart as a convenience.

Breakfast

Banana Toast with Peanut Butter

- 1 Tbsp. of salted peanut butter = 3
- 1 slice of whole wheat bread = 2
- 1 cup strawberries – sliced = 0
- 1 small banana – sliced =0

Smart Points: 5

Snack

- 1 cup blueberries = 0
- 10 chopped peanuts = 2
- 1/2 cup light vanilla yogurt = 1

Lunch

Turkey Sandwich with Chipotle Mayo

- 1 tablespoon light mayonnaise = 2
- 1/8 teaspoon table salt = 0
- Canned chipotle peppers in adobo sauce, minced = 0
- Deli-sliced turkey (2 ounces), smoked variety = 1
- Rye bread - 2 slices reduced-calorie, toasted if desired = 3
- Hass avocado - 1/4 item, mashed = 2
- Plum tomato - 1 medium, cut into 4 slices = 0

1 apple = 0
Mini pretzels - 1 serving = 3
Smart Points: Eight

Snack

- Carrot and celery sticks = 0
- Bean dip: 1/4 cup fat-free = 1

Dinner
- **Farmers Casserole**
- *Plus (+) 7 Per Serving*:

Dessert

Chocolate Raspberry "S'mores"
- 2 graham cracker squares = 2
- 12 mini marshmallows = 1
- A few fresh raspberries = 0
- 1 tablespoon light chocolate syrup = 1

Smart Points: Four

Chapter 2: The Thirty Day Plan

Each of these menu plans is your key to the future of weight loss. If you follow these as shown in the following chapters with the provided Weight Watchers counts provided for each of the delicious meals. You will notice an asterisk (*) next to the menu items as well as the points for each one; these are the ones which have recipes included in the enclosed chapters.

Day 1

- **Eggs Benedict ***
  Points per Serving: +5

- **Cherry-Waldorf Salad***
  6 Smart Points per Serving

- **Roasted Sirloin Beef ***
  4 Points Plus Value per Serving

Day 2

- **Strawberry-Oatmeal Smoothie ***
  4 Smart Points per Serving

- **Quinoa Black Bean Salad ***
  5 Smart Points per Serving

- **Roasted Sirloin Beef ***
  Points Plus Value of 4 per Serving

Day 3

- **BLT Wraps ***
  3 Smart Points per Serving

- **Beef and Pinto Bean Chili ***
  8 Points Plus Value Per Serving

- **Chicken Marsala** *
  4 Points per Serving

Day 4

- **Strawberry Blender Muffins** *
  5 Smart Points per Serving

- **Tuna Salad & Stuffed Tomatoes** *
  Points + Per Serving: Value 4

- **Chicken Fried Steaks** *
  6 Smart Points per Serving

Day 5

- **Egg Muffins** *
  5 Smart Points per Serving

- **Chicken Spinach Crescent Ring** *
  3 Points per Serving

- **Crab Cake Burgers** *
  4 Points (+) Per Serving (Not counting the buns)

Day 6

- **Breakfast Pizza***
  Plus + Six (6) per Serving

- **Quinoa and Tomato Salad** *
  5 Point Plus Value per Serving

- **Tilapia Parmesan** *
  6 Points per Serving

Day 7

- **Steak and Eggs (WW Style) ***
  Smart Points per Serving: 2

- **Arabic Fattoush Salad ***
  2 Smart Points per Serving

- **Lemon Parmesan Chicken Piccata ***
  Smart Points per Serving: 6

Day 8

- **Cheese and Fruit 'Danish' ***
  5 Points plus Value per Serving

- **Spinach and Cheddar Frittata ***
  3 Points plus Value per Serving

- **Shrimp with a Spicy Sauce ***
  2 Points per Serving

Day 9

- **Pumpkin Pie Smoothie ***
  4 Points Plus per Serving

- **WW Cabbage Soup ***
  Zero Points Plus Value Per Serving

- **Beef and Pinto Bean Chili ***
  8 Points Plus Value Per Serving

Day 10

- **Mexican Scrambled Egg Sandwiches**
  Points Plus Value: 5

- **Italian Avocado Salad ***

4 Points per Serving

- **Grilled Pineapple Halibut ***
  Smart Points per Serving: Four

Day 11

- **Yogurt −Fruit & Cereal Sundae ***
  6 Points Plus Value per Serving

- **General TSO's Chicken ***
  8 Smart Points; 8 Points Plus; 7 POINTS (old)

- **Sautéed Spinach and Garlic ***
  2 Points plus Value per Serving

Day 12

- **Cherry-Waldorf Salad ***
  6 Smart Points per Serving

- **Grilled Chicken ***
  4 Points Plus Per Serving

- **Cheesy Cauliflower Bake ***
  Plus+ 4 per Serving

Day 13

- **Corn Quiche ***
  4 Smart Points/4 Points +

- **Summertime Veggie Soup ***
  Plus (+) 3 per Serving

- **Baked Pork Cutlets**
  Plus+ 5 Points per Serving

Day 14

- **Blueberry & Peach Stuffed French Toast ***
  4 Points Value

- **Pizza Pasta Salad ***
  6 Smart Points per Serving

- **Asian Salisbury Steaks ***
  Plus+ 7 per Serving

Day 15

- **Monkey Shake ***
  3 Points+ per Serving

- **Angel Hair Pasta & Eggplant ***
  Smart Points per Serving: 6

- **Stuffed Cabbage Leaves**
  Plus+ 6 per Serving

Day 16

- **Ricotta – Blueberry Buttermilk Pancakes ***
  4 Smart Points

- **Quinoa and Tomato Salad ***
  5 Point Plus Value per Serving

- **Stuffed Cabbage Leaves (leftovers)**

Day 17

- **Green Smoothie**
  5 Points +

- **Layered BLT Salad**
  Plus+ 4 per Serving

- **Ham and Noodle Casserole**
  Plus+ 5 per Serving

Day 18

- **Good Morning Wrap**
  Plus+ 6 per Serving

- **Chicken Noodle Soup (WW Style) ***
  5 Smart Points; 5 Points Plus; 4 Points (old) Per Serving

- **Quinoa Black Bean Salad ***
  5 Smart Points per Serving

Day 19

- **Dutch Babies (Pancake Type) ***
  Each serving = 5 Smart Points/5 Points +

- **Chicken Taco Salad ***
  Each Serving: 7 Smart Points; 8 Points Plus; 6 points
(old)

- **Filet Mignon & Caramelized Onions**
  7 Points+ per Serving

Day 20

- **Kiwi & Banana Salad***
  Points Plus + 5 per Serving

- **Baked Ziti***
  Points: Plus+ 7 per Serving

- **Baked Parmesan Fish**
  Points Plus+ 4 per Serving

Day 21

- **Ham and Swiss in the Skillet**
  6 Smart Points; 6 Points Plus; 5 Points (old system)

- **Philly Cheese Steaks** *
  7 Points (old) (For one serving)

- **Shrimp Scampi** *
  Plus+ 4 per Serving

Day 22

- **Cracking Chicken Slaw** *
  2 Smart Points per Serving

- **Broiled Scallops**
  Smart Points: 6 per Serving

Day 23

- **Cocoa-Nut Bananas** *
  Plus + 2 Points per Serving

- **Pork Barbecue Sandwiches with Coleslaw** *
  6 Points per serving

- **Chicken Teriyaki & Broccoli** *
  Points Plus Value: 7 per Serving

Day 24

- **Berry Breakfast Smoothie***
  Plus+ 4 per Serving

- **French Bread Pizza Caprese**
  7 Smart Points

- **Ranch Meatballs** *
  4 Smart Points/ 5 Points+ per Serving

Day 25

- **Peanut Butter Cup Smoothie** *
  Plus+ 5 for each serving

- **Chicken Fettuccine** *
  3 Points per Serving

- **Zucchini Carpaccio**
  2 Smart Points

Day 26

- **Home-Style Pancakes**
  6 Smart Points; 6 Points Plus; 5 Points (old system) per Serving

- **Lime-Honey Salmon** *
  5 Smart Points per Serving

- **Spaghetti Carbonara** *
  6 Smart Points; 6 Points Plus per Serving

Day 27

- **Ham and Swiss in the Skillet**
  Plus+ 6 per Serving

- **Buffalo Chicken Wings** *
  3 Points + per Serving

- **Sautéed Tomatoes and Cauliflower** *
  Points + per Serving: Value 2

- **Mexican Chicken Breasts** *
  4 Points per Serving

Day 28

- **Kiwi-Banana Smoothie**
  4 Points Plus per Serving

- **Baked Tuna Melt***
  Smart Points/6 Points Plus - per serving

- **Balsamic & Raspberry Chicken ***
  5 Smart Points; 4 Points Plus; 4 POINTS (old)

Day 29

- **Sunrise Smoothie ***
  Plus+ 4 per Serving

- **Tuscan Pasta ***
  Plus+ 5 per Serving

- **Crab Quesadillas ***
  9 Smart Points; 8 Points Plus; 6 Points (old)

Day 30

- **Spiced Cinnamon Apple Oatmeal ***
  6 Points+ /Smart Points 7

- **Skirt Steak with Romesco Sauce ***
  5 Points plus Value per Serving

- **Maple Glazed Salmon ***
  7 Smart Points per Serving

Chapter 3: Rejuvenating Breakfast Recipes

As a quick note about the following recipes; you may notice some of the items are 'divided' which means the ingredient mentioned will be used in more than one place in the recipe. Also, in most recipes where olive oil is listed; it is for extra-virgin olive oil.

Eggs Benedict*

Ingredients
1 tsp. Dijon mustard
2 tsp. skim milk
3 Tbsp. Sour cream
2 eggs
2-ounces reduced-sodium cooked ham (thinly sliced)
1 English muffin (whole wheat) sliced in half
2 Slices of tomato
Optional: Fresh chives

Instructions
1) Heat the broiler in the oven. Preheat a lightly greased medium-sized skillet.
2) *Make the Sauce*: Blend the mustard, milk, and sour cream; set to the side.
3) Halfway fill the prepared skillet with water. Let it boil, and lower the heat to a simmer.
4) Crack one of the eggs into a container and slide it into the water.
5) Hold the eggs as close to the water before releasing as possible.
6) Leave the skillet uncovered and continue to simmer the eggs for three to five minutes. The yolks don't need to be hard, but the whites should be set.
7) In the meantime; put the cut side up of the muffin onto a cookie sheet.
8) Broil three to four inches from the heat source for about one or two minutes to the desired crispness.
9) Top them off with tomato and ham slices. Broil until the toppings are warmed—usually about one minute.

10) Take the eggs out of the skillet and put them on top of the muffin.
11) Garnish with some chives and enjoy.

Points per Serving: +5
Yields: Two Servings

Good Morning Wrap *

Ingredients
2 t. olive oil
¼ t. black pepper
1 green pepper (finely chopped)
2 C. fresh sliced mushrooms
1 C. cholesterol-free egg product
½ C. chunky salsa (your favorite)
4 (Eight-inch) flour tortillas

Instructions
1) Prepare the veggies in a fry pan using medium heat. Pour the oil into the frying pan and simmer them for three to four minutes.
2) Add the black pepper and egg product—mixing well—cooking for three to five minutes.
3) Pour in the salsa and simmer for two minutes on low heat—stir occasionally.

Plus+ 6 per Serving
Yields: Four Servings

Ham and Swiss in the Skillet *

Ingredients
3 Tablespoons (divided) grated Parmesan cheese
1 C. 1% milk (low-fat)
2 Tablespoons all-purpose flour
½ C. light shredded Cheddar cheese
¼ teaspoon hot pepper sauce
½ teaspoon spicy brown mustard
2 sliced tomatoes
½ Pound sliced turkey breast

4 slices light whole grain bread
4 slices turkey bacon (cut in half and cooked)

Instructions

1) *Make the Sauce*: Pour the flour and milk into a small pan stirring until the sauce begins to boil and get thicker
2) Reduce the heat setting and sauté for about three minutes.
3) Take away from the heat, and blend the 2 tablespoons of Parmesan cheese, cheddar cheese, hot pepper sauce, and the mustard. Set it aside.

4) *Prepare the Sandwiches*: Cook the turkey bacon in a skillet and set to the side. Warm up the broiler on the oven.
5) Toast the bread—arranging it on the bottom of four individual ovenproof containers.
6) Place the slices of tomato, the turkey breast, and some of the sauce over each one. Sprinkle the remainder of the cheese onto the upmost layer of the sandwiches.
7) Put them in the oven for a short time about five inches from the heat source.
8) Take them from the oven and place a strip of bacon on each hot sandwich.

6 Smart Points; 6 Points Plus; 5 Points (old system)
Yields: Six Servings (one sandwich for each)
Preparation Time: Five minutes
Cooking time: Fifteen minutes

BLT Wraps *

Ingredients
2 slices fat-free bacon
1 large stone-ground 100% whole wheat tortilla
½ cup chopped romaine lettuce
5 halved grape tomatoes
1 tablespoon Monterey Jack cheese (grated)
1 teaspoon ranch dressing

Instructions
1) Use a skillet to fry/prepare the bacon according to the manufacturer's directions.
2) Warm the tortilla and place a layer of dressing on its top.
3) When the bacon has finished cooking; chop it into small crunchy pieces.
4) Put the lettuce and tomatoes in the center and add the bacon.
5) Garnish with the remainder of the ingredients.
6) Roll and serve.

3 Smart Points per Serving
Yields: One Serving

Mexican Scrambled Egg Sandwiches *

Ingredients
6 Large eggs + an additional four egg whites
3 T. uncooked sliced scallion
2 T. fresh cilantro (chopped)
1/8 tsp. ground black pepper
½ tsp. table salt
6 light English muffins
¾ cups fat-free salsa (chunky style)
2 sprays cooking spray

Directions
1) Prepare a heavy-duty pan with some spray using med-high heat on the stovetop.
2) Whisk the egg whites, eggs, cilantro, salt, pepper, and scallions in a mixing bowl.
3) Empty the eggs into the heated skillet and scramble about 2 ½ minutes. The egg will be slightly moist—but don't overcook.
4) Take the eggs off of the burner and blend in the salsa.
5) Divide the eggs into each of the muffins.

Points Plus Value: 5
Yields: Six Servings (One Sandwich per serving)
Preparation Time: Ten minutes: Cook time: Three minutes

Steak and Eggs (WW Style) *

Ingredients
Cooking spray
4 large eggs and 4 egg whites
2 Tablespoons club soda
1/8 teaspoon each:
- Salt
- Pepper

8 ounces deli-style roast beef slices (thick cut)
3 Tablespoons steak sauce

Instructions
1) Grease a skillet with the cooking spray and put it on the stovetop using the medium heat setting.
2) Blend the club soda, egg whites, and eggs in a mixing container. Empty into the heated pan, cooking until one side is firm.
3) Fold into an omelet and cook for two to three minutes. Take them from the pan and set them to the side in a warming dish.
4) Place the beef into the pan—flipping once—cook for one to two minutes.
5) Slice into quarters and flavor with the pepper and salt with 2 ounces of roast beef and 2 ¼ teaspoons of your favorite steak sauce.

Note: You can substitute 'steak' for the roast beef, but you will need to adjust the Smart Points values.
Yields: Four Servings
Prep Times: 7 minutes; *Cooking Time*: 8 minutes

Corn Quiche *

This tasty quiche takes a little more than thirty minutes, but it is so good. You could cook it the night before and warm it up on the way out of the door! Or, enjoy it on the weekend when you have a little extra time.

Ingredients
1 C. liquid egg substitute

½ C. shredded cheddar cheese (reduced-fat)
1- Can (15-oz.) Corn (drained)
1 C. - 2% milk
1 tsp. onion powder
¼ C. whole wheat flour
1 tsp. baking powder

Instructions
1) Set the oven temperature to 375°F. Prepare a baking dish/pie pan with some cooking spray.
2) Mix all of the ingredients listed (omit 1/2 of the corn) into a blender—mixing until well combined.
3) Add the remainder of corn and stir.
4) Pour the mixture into a baking dish.
5) Bake for approximately 35 minutes until the center comes out clean when tested with a toothpick.
6) Let it rest a few minutes before slicing into six pieces.

4 Smart Points/4 Points +
Yields: Six Servings
Prep Times: Ten minutes; *Cooking Time*: Thirty-five minutes

Breakfast Pizza *

Ingredients
1 Minced garlic clove
1 ½ C. frozen hash browns with onions and peppers (diced and loosely packed)
6 beaten eggs/1 ½ cups frozen or refrigerated egg product
1 Tbsp. Fresh basil (snipped)
1/3 C. fat-free milk
½ tsp. salt
1-ounce Italian bread shell (Boboli)
2 halved plum tomatoes
1 Tbsp. Olive oil
1 C. (4-ounces) shredded mozzarella cheese (part-skim)
¼ C. fresh shredded basil
¼ tsp. ground black pepper

Instructions
1) Set the temperature in the oven to 375°F.

2) Slice the tomatoes lengthwise and as well as sliced into small pieces for the pie.
3) Over the stovetop, using the medium heat setting, prepare a large frying pan with some cooking spray—add the oil.
4) Toss in the garlic and potatoes—cooking until the veggies are tender which is usually for approximately four minutes.

5) In a small mixing container, whisk the freshly snipped basil, the egg, pepper, and salt. Empty the egg mixture into the prepared pan until the egg begins to cook around the edges. Lift and fold the egg mix using a large spatula—continuing until done. Take the pan off of the burner.
6) Assemble the breakfast pizza with the shell on a 12-inch pan or a baking sheet. Layer the cheese, egg, tomatoes, and finish with the top layer of cheese.
7) Bake for ten minutes or until it is ready for your plate.
8) Garnish with some of the fresh basil.

Plus + Six (6) per Serving
Yields: Eight Servings

Egg Muffins *

Ingredients
1 Green bell pepper
15 Large eggs
1 Cup low-fat shredded cheddar cheese
Garlic seasoning (to taste)
Optional: ¼ cup feta cheese

Instructions
1) Heat the oven to 375°F. If you are using muffin tins; use two liners or spray a pan with a cooking spray.
2) Whisk the eggs; add the cheese and veggies along with the garlic seasoning.
3) Empty the mix into tins up to 2/3 full.
4) Bake 25 to 35 minutes until the muffins rise—brown—and set.

You can freeze these and reheat or keep in the refrigerator for one week.
Microwave the muffins for two minutes on the high setting to reheat.

5 Smart Points per Serving
Yields: 12 Servings (1 egg muffin each serving)
Cooking Time: 25-30 minutes

Spinach and Cheddar Frittata *

Ingredients
1 spray cooking spray
1 C. Fresh baby spinach (chopped)
2 large egg whites & 4 Large eggs
2 Tbsp. Uncooked finely chopped scallions
¼ tsp. each:
- Table salt
- Black pepper

1 spray cooking spray
½ C. shredded cheddar cheese (semi-soft & fat-free)

Instructions
1) Heat the oven to 400°F. Coat a twelve-inch skillet (oven-proof) with the puff of cooking spray. Preheat the pan using the medium heat setting.
2) Combine the egg whites and eggs in a large mixing container; blend the scallion, salt, spinach, and pepper into the eggs.
3) Empty the eggs into the hot skillet and cook about five minutes or until partially set. Sprinkle them with the cheese.
4) Place in the oven for about five minutes. Take them out and let it rest for one minute and cut it into eight wedges.

3 Points plus Value per Serving
Yields: Four Servings (2 wedges each)
Prep Time: Twelve minutes; *Cooking Time*: Ten minutes

Pancakes

Home-Style Pancakes

Ingredients
1/3 C. Unsweetened applesauce
¾ C. whole wheat flour
½ T. baking powder
1 lightly beaten egg white
½ C. skim/fat-free buttermilk
½ teaspoon cinnamon
Options: No sweeteners
    Or 1 to 2 teaspoons of artificial sweetener

Instructions
1) Combine the sweetener (if used), cinnamon, flour, applesauce, buttermilk, egg, and baking powder until the mixture is creamy smooth.
2) *Note*: You can add a small amount of water if the mixture is too thick (only about one Tbsp. at a time).
3) Prepare a large griddle or skillet and coat it with a squirt of butter-flavored cooking oil.
4) Place about two heaping tablespoons of the pancake batter onto the heated skillet. When the bubbles form—flip them and cook for about one more minute.
5) What a treat! Adjust the ingredients and points to accommodate your crowd.

6 Smart Points; 6 Points Plus; 5 Points (old system) per Serving
Yields: Two Servings
Preparation Time is ten minutes.
Cooking Time is also ten minutes.

Dutch Babies (Pancake Type) *

Ingredients
4 eggs
1 C. skim milk
½ tsp. salt
1 C. all-purpose/gluten-free flour

25

4 Tbsp. butter (divided & melted)

Instructions
1) Heat the oven in advance to 400°F.
2) Prepare a 13x9-inch pan/dish with 2 T. of butter. Place the baking dish in the oven to melt the butter.
3) Use the blender to whip the eggs until fluffy—for about thirty to sixty seconds.
4) Blend in the remainder of the ingredients and mix for an additional minute—until combined.
5) Empty the batter mixture into the pan and bake for eighteen to twenty minutes.
6) Garnish with your favorite toppings. (Be sure to add the points, if any.)

Each Serving = 5 Smart Points/5 Points +
Yields: Six Servings
Prep Time: 5 minutes plus oven preheat cycle: Cook time: 20 minutes

Ricotta – Blueberry Buttermilk Pancakes *

This recipe is an excellent vegetarian dish.

Ingredients
1/3 cup water
1 cup whole wheat buttermilk pancake mix
½ teaspoon nutmeg (freshly grated)
1 teaspoon each
- Vanilla extract
- Lemon juice
- Freshly grated lemon zest

½ cup each
- Liquid egg substitute
- Part-skim ricotta cheese
- Fresh/frozen blueberries

Instructions
1) Prepare a skillet with some non-fat butter flavored cooking spray.
2) Blend the flour and nutmeg in a small dish.

3) Mix the lemon juice, lemon zest, vanilla extract, egg substitute, and ricotta in a large mixing container until it's creamy.
4) Blend the ingredients until you reach the desired consistency. You may need to add a small amount of water.
5) Using medium heat, empty some of the batter in the prepared pan to make two to four pancakes—sprinkle the blueberries—and cook for two minutes. When you see the air bubbles—turn them—cooking for another two minutes or until nicely browned.

4 Smart Points
Yields: (Serving size is two pancakes)
Prep Time is five minutes with an additional five minutes for cooking.

Blueberry & Peach Stuffed French Toast *

Ingredients
1 C. frozen/thawed peaches or 1 large peach chopped
1 C. fresh/frozen/thawed blueberries
16-Slices whole wheat light bread
2 ½ C. Fat-free skim milk
1 Tbsp. Powdered sugar
2-C. egg substitute (fat-free)
2 Tbsp. Granulated sugar
One tsp. Each:
- Cinnamon
- Vanilla extract

Instructions
1) Heat the oven temperature to 400°F.
2) Use a 13 x 9 baking dish and position about half of the slices in one layer.
3) Sprinkle the peaches and blueberries over the top of the bread.
4) In a medium mixing container, blend the egg substitute, milk, sugar, vanilla extract, and cinnamon.

5) Pour half of the mix over the fruit and place a layer of bread. Empty the remaining contents over the bread while pressing the 'sandwich' together.
6) Place a cover on the dish and bake for twenty minutes.
7) Uncover and let it cook about ten more minutes.
8) Cool slightly and enjoy!

4 Points Value
Yields: Eight Servings
Cook time: 30 minutes

Chapter 4: The Sweeter Side of Breakfast

Smoothies and Yogurt

Berry Breakfast Smoothie *

You can use the berries of your choice; such as blackberries, raspberries, strawberries, or blueberries.

Ingredients
1 ¼ cups of berries
1/2 cup plain yogurt (low-fat)
1 banana
1 ¼ Cup Orange juice
Optional: 1 Tablespoon Splenda® Granular

Instructions
1) Combine all of the ingredients using a blender until your smoothie is creamy smooth.
2) Serve right away.

Plus+ 4 per Serving
Yields: Three Servings (One cup each)

Green Smoothie *

Ingredients
One Cup each:
- Coconut water
- Kale
- Spinach
- Plain non-fat yogurt
- Frozen mango

1 Pear
Optional: ¼ teaspoon vanilla extract

Instructions
1) Use a blender and mix all of the ingredients until creamy smooth.
2) Serve cold.

5 Points +
Yields: Two Servings (12-Ounce Servings)

Kiwi-Banana Smoothie *

Ingredients
½ Cup ice cubes
1- Kiwi fruit (1/2 Cup)
1 banana
1 Cup low-fat yogurt
Optional: 2 teaspoons maple syrup

Instructions
1) Peel and cut the Kiwi fruit and banana into chunks.
2) Blend everything on the list until smooth and serve immediately.

Yields: Two Servings
4 Points Plus per Serving

Monkey Shake *

Ingredients
1 Fully ripe banana
2 C. fat-free milk
1 - Package JELL-O® (1.4-ounces)
        Fat-free Chocolate/Sugar-free Instant Pudding
Last Step: 2 C. crushed ice

Instructions
1) Cut the banana into chunks.
2) Mix all of the listed ingredients (omit the ice) in a blender and mix well.
3) Add the ice, and blend using the high speed until it is creamy smooth.
4) Enjoy as a super quick breakfast or any other time of day!

3 Points+ per Serving
Yields: Four (1-cup servings)

Peanut Butter Cup Smoothie *

Ingredients
1 C. Chocolate 1% low-fat milk
1 C. ripe sliced banana
½ C. vanilla frozen yogurt (low-fat)
1 - Carton vanilla low-fat yogurt (8-ounces)
2 tablespoons peanut butter (natural-style)

Instructions
1) Freeze the banana in the freezer for about one hour.
2) Take it out and let it stand for about five minutes.
3) Combine all of the ingredients on the list in a blender and work it until the shake is creamy smooth.

Plus+ 5 for each serving
Yields: Three Servings (one cup each)

Pumpkin Pie Smoothie *

Ingredients
1 Tablespoon honey
½ Cup each:
- Vanilla soy milk
- Canned pumpkin
- Crushed ice

1 teaspoon pumpkin pie spice

Instructions
1) Blend all of the ingredients together and serve.

4 Points Plus per Serving
Yields: One Serving

Berry Breakfast Smoothie *

You can use the berries of your choice; such as blackberries, raspberries, strawberries, or blueberries.

Ingredients
1 ¼ cups of berries

1 banana
1/2 cup low-fat plain yogurt or you may choose the low-fat silken tofu
1 ¼ Cup Orange juice
Optional Ingredient: 1 Tablespoon Splenda® Granular

Instructions
1) Combine all of the ingredients using a blender until your smoothie is creamy smooth.
2) Serve right away.

Plus+ 4 per Serving
Yields: Three Servings (One cup each)

Green Smoothie *

Ingredients
One Cup each:
- Coconut water
- Kale
- Spinach
- Plain non-fat yogurt
- Frozen mango

1 Pear
Optional: ¼ teaspoon vanilla extract

Instructions
1) Use a blender and mix all of the ingredients until creamy smooth.
2) Serve cold.

5 Points +
Yields: Two Servings (12-Ounce Servings)

Kiwi-Banana Smoothie *

Smoothie Ingredients
1 kiwifruit (1/2 Cup)
1 banana
1 Cup low-fat yogurt
½ Cup ice cubes

Optional: 2 teaspoons maple syrup

Instructions
Peel and cut the kiwifruit and bananas into chunks.
Combine everything on the list until smooth and serve
immediately.

Yields: Two Servings
4 Points Plus per Serving

Monkey Shake *

Ingredients
1 Fully ripe banana
2 Cups fat-free milk
1 - Package (1.4-ounces) Fat-free Chocolate/Sugar-free Instant
Pudding
2 Cups crushed ice

Instructions
1) Cut the banana into chunks.
2) Combine everything on the list of ingredients (omit the
   ice) in a blender mixing well.
3) Add the ice, and blend using the high speed until it is
   creamy smooth.
4) Enjoy as a super quick breakfast or any other time of day!

3 Points+ per Serving
Yields: Four (1-cup servings)

Peanut Butter Cup Smoothie *

Ingredients
1 C. Chocolate 1% low-fat milk
1 C. ripe sliced banana
½ C. vanilla frozen yogurt (low-fat)
1 (8-ounce) carton vanilla yogurt (low-fat)
2 Tbsp. Peanut butter (natural-style)

Instructions
1) Freeze the banana in the freezer for about one hour.

2) Take it out and let it stand for about five minutes.
3) In a blender, mix all of the ingredients until the shake is creamy smooth.

Plus+ 5 for each serving
Yields: Three Servings (one cup each)

Pumpkin Pie Smoothie *

Ingredients
1 Tablespoon honey
½ Cup each:
- Vanilla soy milk
- Canned pumpkin
- Crushed ice
1 teaspoon pumpkin pie spice

Instructions
1) Blend all of the ingredients together and serve.

4 Points Plus per Serving
Yields: One Serving

Strawberry-Oatmeal Smoothie *

Ingredients
2 scoops protein powder (unsweetened/30 g protein per scoop)
½ cup instant oatmeal
1 cup frozen strawberries
1 medium banana
1 ½ cups skim milk
Optional: ¼ teaspoon vanilla

Instructions
1) Use a blender to combine all of the ingredients until creamy smooth.
2) Refrigerate or serve right away.

4 Smart Points per Serving
Yields: Four Servings
Prep Time: Five minutes

Sunrise Smoothie *

Ingredients
1 container low-fat vanilla yogurt
1 small banana
1 cup whole strawberries
1 cup ice
4 ounces low-calorie orange soda
Note: Sunkist is a good choice.
Instructions
   1) Cut the banana into chunks.
   2) Add the yogurt to the blender—followed by the banana—blending until smooth.
   3) Add the soda—blend—then the ice—and blend until creamy smooth.

Plus+ 4 per Serving
Yields: Two Servings

Yogurt –Fruit & Cereal Sundae *

Ingredients
½ cup chopped strawberries
1 cup fat-free Greek yogurt (plain)
½ of a large biscuit of shredded wheat (12.5 grams)
1 Cup fat-free latte (no sugar)

Instructions
   1) Use the berries to garnish the yogurt and crumble the wheat over the top.
   2) For additional flavor add some almond extract or ground cinnamon.

6 Points Plus Value per Serving
Yields: One serving
Prep Time: 5 Minutes; *Cooking Time*: Zero

Cheese and Fruit Danish *

Ingredients
8 ounces of black coffee
2 slices wheat bread (reduced-calorie)
½ cup each:
- Fresh blueberries
- Fat-free ricotta cheese

½ teaspoon sugar substitute
¼ teaspoon cinnamon

Optional Garnishes for Flavor Boosts
- Fresh mint
- Lemon zest
- Ground nutmeg

Instructions
1) Toast the bread and spread with ¼ cup of the berries and ¼ cup of the ricotta.
2) Blend the cinnamon with the sugar substitute and sprinkle the top.
3) Broil until the berries begin to burst

Have a nice cup of coffee to complement the meal.

Substitutes: You can begin with thin sandwich bread or an English muffin and top with a thinly sliced apple, pear or banana. Be sure to compensate for the points when you choose your toppings.

5 Points plus Value per Serving
Yields: One Serving
Prep Time: Five minutes
Cooking time: Zero

Cocoa-Nut Bananas *

Ingredients
2 bananas (sliced diagonally
4 Teaspoons Each:
- Unsweetened Coconut
- Cocoa Powder

Instructions
1) Put the coconut and cocoa in a separate container.
2) Roll each of the bananas into cocoa first—shake the excess away.
3) Dip it into the coconut. Enjoy the tasty treat.

Plus + 2 Points per Serving
Yields: Four Servings

Spiced Cinnamon Apple Oatmeal *

Ingredients
2 Tablespoons apple butter
1/3 cup uncooked quick oats
1 Tablespoon low-fat granola
Dash of cinnamon
Optional: Splash of skim milk

Instructions
1) Prepare the oats according to the label directions.
2) Blend in the cinnamon, granola, and apple butter.
Yields: One serving
6 Points+ /Smart Points 7

Strawberry Blender Muffins *

Ingredients
2 Lg. Bananas
2 C. oats
2 Large eggs
1 ½ t. baking powder
1 C. plain non-fat yogurt
½ - teaspoon each:
- Vanilla extract
- Baking soda
1/8 t. salt
2C. fresh strawberries

Instructions
1) Heat the oven to 400°F.

2) Use a small amount of cooking spray to spray the muffin pan/tin and place some paper liners in the cup. Set to the side.
3) Use a food processor/blender to mix the eggs, yogurt, salt, vanilla, baking soda, baking powder, oats, and bananas. Process/blend until creamy smooth. Toss and fold in the berries.
4) Empty the batter evenly into the tins and bake for fifteen to twenty minutes.
5) Cool about 10 minutes or so and enjoy.

5 Smart Points per Serving
Yields: 12 muffins: 1 each for the count
Prep Time: Seven Minutes
Cooking Time: Twenty Minutes

Chapter 5: Satisfying Salads and Soups Recipes

Arabic Fattoush Salad *

Ingredients
Pepper and Salt
1- Whole wheat pita bread
2 cups halved grape tomatoes
1 large diced English* cucumber (about 2 cups)
½ medium finely diced red onion
2 cups grape tomatoes (cut into halves)
¾ cup each:
- Fresh Mint leaves
- Fresh Chopped Parsley

1-minced garlic clove
Juice of ½ Lemon
1 tablespoon olive oil
1/4 cup fat-free feta cheese
1 teaspoon ground sumac

Instructions
1) Finely chop the parsley and mint leaves.
2) Mist the pita bread with a bit of salt and cooking spray.
3) Toast it until brown and chop it into small bite-sized pieces.
4) Toss the remainder of ingredients in a large bowl—OMIT the feta.
5) Use the diced feta cheese and pita for the garnish.

2 Smart Points per Serving
Yields: Four Servings
Prep Time: Fifteen minutes

Note: Choose English cucumbers which are seedless and longer than the typical variety. They are also called greenhouse or hothouse cucumbers.

Quinoa Black Bean Salad *

Ingredients
Juice of 1 lime
1 minced garlic clove
1 Tablespoon olive oil
Pepper and salt (to taste)
1/3 cup finely chopped cilantro
1 cup uncooked quinoa
1 can black beans (15-ounces)

Instructions
1) Rinse the beans thoroughly and drain them in a colander.
2) Prepare the quinoa according to the directions on the package.
3) Empty them when done into a medium-sized container to cool for approximately ten minutes.
4) Combine the remainder of the ingredients—toss them to blend well.
5) Serve the tasty treat at room temperature.

5 Smart Points per Serving
Yields: Six Servings
Prep Time: Five minutes; *Cook time*: Fifteen minutes

Quinoa and Tomato Salad *

Ingredients
2 C. grape or cherry tomatoes or any mixture
1 cup uncooked quinoa
1 Tablespoon each
   • White wine vinegar
   • Olive oil
½ teaspoon table salt
2 Tablespoons minced fresh chives
¼ teaspoon black pepper

Instructions
1) Place the quinoa under running water using a fine strainer/mesh sieve until the water is clear. Drain it well.

2) Put the quinoa into a pan of cold water placing it over high heat until it boils.
3) Lower the temperature setting and simmer about 15 minutes.
4) Take it off of the burner, and let it rest for five minutes. After that, spoon out the quinoa and put it into a large container—setting it to the side to cool.
5) In the meantime, reserve two tablespoons of the tomato juice and chop the tomatoes into a fine consistency and set them to the side.
6) Blend in the tomato juice and combine the pepper, salt, and vinegar using a glass cup.
7) Stir it all together and toss. Drizzle with the vinaigrette from step 6.

5 Point Plus Value per Serving
Yields: Four Servings (Approximately 1 ¼ cup)
Preparation Time: Ten minutes; *Actual Cooking Time*: Eighteen minutes

Something Sweet for Lunch

Cherry-Waldorf Salad *

Ingredients
2 large apples
2 chopped celery ribs
1 Tablespoon fresh lemon juice
1 C. pitted sweet cherries
½ C. slivered – toasted almonds
½ C. dried Cranberries
¼ C. each:
   • Light sour cream
   • Light mayonnaise
1/8 teaspoon salt
2 Tablespoons honey

Instructions
1) Fuji apples work best and should be cored and chopped.
2) Prepare the salad - beginning with combining the apples and the lemon juice in a big salad serving bowl.

3) Toss in the cherries, celery, almonds, and cranberries.
4) Using a small dish, whisk the sour cream, mayonnaise, salt, and honey until well combined.
5) Cover the bowl and refrigerate a minimum of 1-hour before mealtime.

Six Smart Points per Serving

Italian Avocado Salad *

Ingredients
1 (2.25 ounce) Can of sliced & drained olives
1 pint (halved) grape tomatoes
1 (18-ounce) bag romaine hearts
1 medium cucumber
1 avocado
¾ cup light Italian dressing

Instructions
1) Peel, pit, and dice the avocado into chunks. Peel (unless you like the peeling), and chop the cucumbers and cut the romaine lettuce while draining the olives.
2) Combine all of the ingredients and sprinkle with the salad dressing.

4 Points per Serving
Yields: Eight Servings (1 ½ Cups each)

Kiwi & Banana Salad

Ingredients
1 Tbsp. Minced shallot
2 tsp. rice vinegar
1 Tbsp. Canola oil
¼ tsp. salt
1 tsp. honey
2 Tbsp. lime juice
A sprinkle of cayenne pepper
2 ripe – firm bananas
4 peeled and diced kiwis
½ C. diced red bell pepper

2 Tbsp. each:
- Chopped cashews
- Fresh Mint (thinly sliced)

Instructions
1) Slice the bananas into ½-inch thick slices, cut diagonally.
2) Whisk the honey, shallot, lime juice salt, cayenne, and vinegar in a mixing container.
3) Toss in the bell peppers, kiwis, mind, and bananas—tossing well.
4) Serve with a sprinkling of cashews.

Points Plus + 5 per Serving
Yields: 4 (1 ½ cup servings)
Prep Time: Twenty minutes
Cooking time: Ten minutes

Soup

Beef and Pinto Bean Chili *

Ingredients
1 medium minced clove garlic
1 pound uncooked ground beef (93% lean)
1 package frozen mixed veggies
1 Can (14 1/2 –ounce) of diced tomatoes with chipotle chilies
2 tsp. chili powder
1 C. fire-roasted canned crushed tomatoes
½ tsp. Table salt
¼ tsp. Crushed dried oregano
1- (15-ounce) Can of pinto beans
¼ tsp. black pepper

Note: For the veggies, you can use some bell peppers mixed with onions.

Instructions
1) Rinse and drain the pinto beans.
2) Prepare the stovetop using the med-high setting. Place a large skillet on the stove prepared with some cooking spray, and add the frozen vegetables along with the garlic—stirring occasionally; usually about three minutes.

Toss in the beef—continue to stir frequently. Cook for about two minutes while you use a wooden spoon to break the chunks of beef.

3) Blend in the crushed and diced tomatoes, chili powder, pepper, salt, beans, and oregano. Turn the heat up to highest setting for approximately three minutes or until it reaches the desired consistency.

8 Points Plus Value Per Serving
Yields: Four Servings (1 ¼ cups for each serving)
Prep Time is fourteen minutes. The *cooking time* is eight minutes.

WW Cabbage Soup *

Ingredients
½ yellow onion
2 minced garlic cloves
3 cups non-fat beef/vegetable/chicken broth
2 cups chopped cabbage
1Tablespoon tomato paste
½ cup each:
- Green beans
- Zucchini
- Carrots

Pepper and Salt
½ teaspoon:
- Oregano
- Basil

Instructions
1) Use some cooking spray in a pot –add the garlic, onions, and carrots and sauté for five minutes.
2) Blend the green beans, cabbage, tomato paste, broth, pepper, salt, oregano, and basil.
3) Simmer the ingredients for about five to ten minutes—toss in the zucchini and continue simmering for about five more minutes.

Zero Points Plus Value Per Serving
Yields: (One cup) Six to Eight Servings

Preparation time is 7 minutes and cooking time is 25 minutes.
Chicken Noodle Soup (WW Style) *

Ingredients
8 ounces chicken breast
1 cup thin spaghetti
5 cups fat-free chicken broth
½ cup each:
- Celery
- Carrots

8 green onions
¼ teaspoon each dried:
- Parsley
- Thyme

A pinch of pepper and salt to taste

Instructions
1) Cut up the chicken into small pieces and chop the celery and carrots. Thinly slice the onion, and break the spaghetti into two-inch pieces.
2) Flavor the chicken with some pepper and salt.
3) On the stovetop, use the medium heat setting, and add some oil to a skillet. Place the chicken and simmer for three to five minutes—stirring constantly.
4) Blend in the remainder of the ingredients to the soup pot until it boils. Lower the heat setting and continue cooking until the spaghetti is the desired consistency.

5 Smart Points; 5 Points Plus; 4 POINTS (old) Per Serving
Yields: Four Servings (1 ¼ cups for each serving)
Prep Time and *cooking time* is 15 minutes each for a total of 30 minutes.

Summertime Veggie Soup *

Ingredients
1 Cup plain Greek chilled yogurt
3 cups chilled & well-shaken buttermilk
2 cups seeded medium tomatoes
2 cups fresh corn kernels
½ cup fresh diced fennel

3 Tablespoons fresh dill (+) more for the garnish
Fresh ground black pepper & kosher salt

Instructions
1) Dice some ripe tomatoes.
2) In a large mixing container, combine the yogurt and buttermilk.
3) Blend in the corn, tomatoes, cucumber, one teaspoon of salt, ¼ teaspoon of pepper, and the fennel.
4) You can serve now, or cover the contents and place in the fridge for up to twenty-four hours.

Plus (+) 3 per Serving
Yields: Eight Servings with about one cup allowed per serving

Chapter 6: Dinner Recipes and Sides
French Bread Pizza Caprese *

Ingredients
1 (8-ounce) whole wheat French bread baquette
2 medium sliced thin tomatoes
4 ounces fresh (sliced thinly) Mozzarella cheese
1 Tablespoon each:
- Fresh chopped basil
- Balsamic glaze

Instructions
1) Slice the bread in half lengthwise—cutting again in half to make four pieces.
2) Place the torn cheese pieces on top of the bread for two to three minutes until the cheese melts.
3) Place on a serving dish, top with the tomatoes, and drizzle some balsamic glaze onto the creation and garnish with a bit of fresh basil.

7 Smart Points
Yields: Four Servings
Total time for prep and cooking is ten minutes.

Filet Mignon & Caramelized Onions *

Ingredients
2 large onions
1 Tablespoon brown sugar
1 Pound fillet Mignon (cut into four steaks—1 ¼-inches thick)
½ cup fat-free beef broth
1 Tablespoon balsamic vinegar
2 Tablespoons light butter
1 teaspoon salt
1/3 cup blue or Gorgonzola cheese
½ teaspoon black pepper (fresh ground)

Instructions
1) In a large heavy-duty pan, melt one tablespoon of butter using medium heat. Combine the brown sugar and onions into the mixture, cooking for about 15 minutes.

2) Pour in the broth along with ½ teaspoon of salt and the vinegar—continue stirring for about three to four minutes. Put the onions in a dish and cover with some foil to keep them warm.
3) Sprinkle the pepper and salt on the steaks for additional flavoring.
4) Using a clean pan, melt the butter using med-high heat. Put the steaks into the hot pan and cook until nicely browned, for three to five minutes.
5) Flip them and top with the cheese, reducing the heat to med-low. Cook three to five minutes if you want a rare steak or longer until it reaches the desired doneness.
6) Combine the onions in the pan to warm and serve. Delicious!

7 Points+ per Serving
Yields: Four Servings (four-ounce servings)
Prep Time: Ten minutes *Cooking Time*: 30 minutes (less if you like it rare)

Roasted Sirloin Beef *

Ingredients
2 Pounds uncooked sirloin beef
Cooking Spray (2 sprays)
4 medium garlic cloves
One tsp. Each:
- Fresh ground black pepper
- Salt
2 Tablespoons each fresh:
- Rosemary
- Oregano

Note: You can substitute two teaspoons each of the oregano and rosemary if you use the dried version.

Instructions
1) Cut away all of the fat from the beef. Mince the garlic cloves, oregano, and rosemary.
2) Heat the oven temperature to 400°F. Prepare a shallow roasting dish with the cooking spray.

3) Add some flavoring to the meat with the salt and pepper.
4) Blend the oregano, rosemary, and garlic in a small mixing container. Rub it over the top of the beef. (Press with your fingertips to be sure it sticks.)
5) Bake approximately 20 minutes until the internal temperature reaches at least 145°F.
6) Before slicing—let the roast rest/sit for five minutes. Slice it against the grain.

Add some Brussels sprouts and roasted potatoes (if you count them for the extra points).

Points Plus of 4 per Serving
Yields: Eight Servings (3 ounces for each serving)
Preparation Time is ten minutes. *Cooking Time* is twenty minutes.

Philly Cheese Steaks *

Ingredients
1 medium yellow onion
1 Pound lean flank steak
1 medium-sized green bell pepper
¼ teaspoon each of salt and pepper
2 teaspoons Worcestershire sauce
4 slices fat-free American cheese
4 high-fiber sandwich rolls

Note: Use a roll listed between 90 to 140 calories each.

Instructions
1) Cut the steak into eight thin slices. Deseed and thinly slice the peppers and onions.
2) Heat the oven to 375°F.
3) Prepare a skillet with some non-fat cooking spray. Sauté the peppers and onions using medium-high heat for approximately ten minutes. Take out of the pan and set to the side.
4) Add the steak—sautéing about one to two minutes on each side.

5) Pour the Worcestershire sauce, pepper, and salt into the pan and simmer until the liquid is completely absorbed.
6) Place the steaks on the buns with the cheese, onions, and peppers.
7) Wrap in some aluminum foil around each sandwich, and put in the oven for five minutes; remove and enjoy!

7 Points (old) (For one serving)
Yields: Four Sandwiches

Skirt Steak with Romesco Sauce *

Ingredients
8 fillets (1 ½ Pounds) thinly sliced skirt steak
1 Jar roasted red peppers (12-ounces)
½ cup grated Parmesan cheese
4 garlic cloves
¼ C. raw almonds
2 Tbsp. balsamic vinegar
½ tsp. black pepper
1 tsp. salt

Directions
1) Drain the red peppers.
2) Heat the grill/grill pan to med-high.
3) Add some additional flavoring to the steak with some pepper and salt.
4) *Grill to your liking:* Three to five minutes per side will provide a medium-rare steak. Let the meat rest/sit for about ten minutes before you slice.
5) Combine the almonds, red peppers, pepper, salt, parmesan cheese, and vinegar in a processor and pulse until smooth.

5 Points plus Value per Serving
Yields: Eight servings (1 serving = 1 fillet with sauce)
Preparation Time: Ten minutes; *Cooking Time*: Ten minutes

Asian Salisbury Steaks *

Ingredients
1 (12-ounce) package 90% Lean ground beef
¾ Cup each:
- Chopped scallions
- Finely diced red bell peppers

¼ Cup Plain breadcrumbs
2 tablespoons fresh minced ginger
4 tablespoons (divided) hoisin sauce
3 teaspoons (divided) canola oil
½ Cup Rice wine or dry sherry
16 cups trimmed watercress/4 bunches/2 (4-ounce) bags

Instructions
1) Heat the broiler and adjust the rack to the upper 1/3 of the oven.
2) Spray the rack and grill pan with cooking spray.
3) Combine the peppers, beef, scallions, ginger, three tablespoons of the hoisin sauce, and breadcrumbs until just combined in a mixing container. Shape four oblong patties and place them on the broiler/pan rack. Use one teaspoon of oil to brush the tops.
4) Place the grill pan in the oven and broil for four minutes on each side.
5) In the meantime, using the stovetop, heat the remainder of the oil in a skillet using the high heat setting.
6) Toss in the watercress and boil one to three minutes or until it begins to wilt. Divvy it up into four serving dishes.
7) Place the skillet, using med-high heat; add the rest of the hoisin sauce and sherry/wine. Blend until bubbly smooth. Lower the heat and cook an additional minute.
8) Top the watercress with the steak and drizzle with the sauce from the pan.

Plus+ 7 per Serving
Yields: Four Servings (1 patty per serving)

Ranch Meatballs *

Ingredients
1/3 Cup panko breadcrumbs

1 Pound Extra-lean ground beef
¼ cup egg substitute (ex. Egg Beaters)
1 Tablespoon each: a. Onion powder; b. Garlic powder
1 tsp. olive oil
2 teaspoons each dried:
- Basil
- Parsley
- Dill

Instructions
1) Combine all of the ingredients by hand (Just like Grandma).
2) Shape into approximately 24 meatballs.
3) Prepare a pan over med-high heat—add the oil.
4) Put the meatballs into the pan and cook for one to two minutes per side until browned.
5) Lower the heat to med-low, and pour in the one-half cup of water.
6) Cover and simmer—occasionally stir—for ten to twelve minutes.

Enjoy just like the ole' folks did long ago.

4 Smart Points/ 5 Points+ per Serving
Yields: Four Servings (Each serving is six meatballs.)
Preparation Time: Ten minutes; *Cooking Time*: Twenty minutes

Stuffed Cabbage Leaves *

Ingredients
2 tablespoons fine dry breadcrumbs
1 Lb. Lean ground beef
1 large head of cabbage
¼ cup each
- Raisins
- Finely chopped onion

1 cup spaghetti sauce
¼ teaspoon ground cinnamon

Instructions
1) Preheat the oven to 350°F.

2) Pull away about twelve of the outer leaves from the head of the cabbage. Also, remove the tough veins from each one. Place them in boiling water for three minutes—drain—continuing until all of the pulled leaves of the cabbage is cooked.

3) Finely chop the remainder of the cabbage (1/2 cup). Keep the remaining section of the cabbage for later use.

4) Using a large skillet, brown the onion and beef, adding the ½ cup of chopped cabbage until the beef is well-done. Drain and stir in the bread crumbs, raisins, and ¼ of the sauce.

5) Scoop ¼ cup (scant) of the mixture on each of the leaves—folding in the sides. Use a two-quart rectangular dish to arrange the rolls.

6) In a small container, mix the cinnamon and spaghetti sauce together and pour over the rolls (reserving some of the liquid for the garnish).

7) Cover the bowl and bake for twenty to twenty-five minutes. Dip the remainder of the sauce over the cabbage rolls and enjoy.

Plus+ 6 per Serving
Yields: Six Servings
Cook time: 20 to 25 minutes

Chicken

Grilled Chicken *

You can compete with "Cracker Barrel" on this one!

Ingredients
1 Pound Chicken breast tenders (deboned & skinless)
1 ½ teaspoons honey
1 teaspoon fresh lime juice
½ cup Italian dressing

Instructions
1) Combine the honey, lime juice, and Italian dressing.

2) Put the tenders into a 'ziploc-type' plastic bag and empty the marinade over the top of the chicken. Place in the fridge for one hour.
3) Use the grill or a skillet to prepare the chicken.
4) Discard the marinade and cook the chicken until it is done and the juice runs clear.

Yields: Two Servings
4 Points Plus Per Serving
It is Ready-to-Serve in 20 minutes.
The preparation time is five minutes.
The cooking time is fifteen minutes.

Balsamic & Raspberry Chicken *

Ingredients
3 chicken breasts (skinless and boneless)
¼ cup all-purpose flour
1 ½ teaspoons cornstarch
Black Pepper and Salt to taste
2/3 cup low-fat chicken broth
1-½ Tablespoons balsamic vinegar
½ Cup low-sugar raspberry preserves

Instructions
1) Slice the chicken up into bite-sized pieces. Flavor each piece with some pepper and salt. Dredge it in flour and shake off the excess.
2) On the stovetop using medium heat, prepare a pan and cook the chicken approximately fifteen minutes—flipping halfway through the cooking process. Take it from the pan and set it to the side.
3) Combine the cornstarch, preserves, and broth over medium heat in the skillet—pour in the vinegar—and place the chicken back into the mixture.
4) Continue cooking for about ten minutes, once again, flipping after about five minutes.

Yields: Four Servings
5 Smart Points; 4 Points Plus; 4 POINTS (old)
Preparation takes ten minutes; ready in 30minutes.

Buffalo Chicken Wings *

Ingredients
12 ounces uncooked chicken wings (skinless)
1 cup hot sauce
1 spray (enough to coat the sheet) Olive oil cooking spray
1 ¼ ounces taco seasoning mix (Old El Paso)
1/2cup fat-free sour cream
2 tablespoons each:
Fat-free skim milk
Gorgonzola or blue cheese (crumbled)
4 medium celery stalks

Directions
1) Set the oven temperature to 400°F.
2) Slice the celery into two-inch pieces.
3) Dip each of the wings into the hot sauce, and place them in a closed zip-lock bag along with the seasonings—shaking to coat.
4) Place on the prepared sheet and bake 18 to 20 minutes.
5) *Prepare the Dip*: Whisk the milk, cheese, and sour cream.
6) Have some dip with celery on the side dish.

3 Points + per Serving
Yields: Four Servings: (1 celery stalk, 3 wings, & 3 tablespoons of dip each)
Cooking Time: Eighteen to Twenty Minutes

Chicken Fettuccine *

Ingredients
1 Package (9-ounce) Refrigerated fresh fettuccine
1 (8-ounce) package broccoli florets/about 4 cups
1/3 Cup honey-Dijon salad dressing (fat-free)
¼ Cup red wine vinegar
1 teaspoon each:
  • Minced garlic
  • Olive oil
¼ teaspoon ground black pepper
1 Tablespoon Dijon mustard
1 (10-ounce) package chicken breasts (no skin or bones)

Or leftover chicken

Instructions
1) Break the pasta in half and prepare according to the directions leaving out any fats and salt. Toss in the broccoli for the last three minutes of the 'pasta' time. Drain and put in a large container.
2) Combine the red wine vinegar, salad dressing, Dijon mustard, garlic, and olive oil. Pour this mixture over your fettuccine and gently toss in the chicken.
3) Garnish with a sprinkle of pepper.

3 Points per Serving
Yields: Eight Servings (One-Cup)
Prep Time: Ten minutes; *Cook Time*: Fifteen minutes

Chicken Fried Steaks *

Ingredients
4 Lean cube steaks
1 cup flour (Reserve 1 Tbsp.)
½ cup Fat-free buttermilk
1 teaspoon each:
- McCormick's Montreal Steak Seasoning
- Salt
2 cups skim milk
2 Tablespoons oil

Instructions
1) Dip each one of the cube steaks into the buttermilk.
2) Blend the steak seasoning (reserving 1 Tbsp.), salt, and flour in a container. Dip each one of the cube steaks into the mixture and place on some sheets of wax paper and let them set for about twenty minutes.
3) In the meantime, on the stovetop, heat one tablespoon of oil in a skillet. Place the steaks into the pan once it is hot—cooking them until they are browned on each side. Take each one out of the pan and place under some foil to keep them warm.
4) Combine the tablespoon of flour and milk until well combined in another bowl. Stir the mixture into the pan

and slowly add the flour mixture until it boils. Lower the heat setting, and let the gravy simmer until it thickens.

6 Smart Points per Serving
Yields: Four Servings (1 Steak for each serving)

Chicken Marsala *

Ingredients
4 boneless thin sliced chicken cutlets/4 chicken breasts
½ teaspoon each
- Ground black pepper
- Salt

2 cups sliced fresh mushrooms
2 teaspoons each:
- All-purpose flour
- Olive Oil

¼ cup each:
- Reduced-sodium chicken broth
- Marsala Wine

Instructions
1) Prepare a skillet on the medium-high setting, with a small amount of oil. Toss in the chicken and cook for three minutes per side. Place it into a container to keep warm.
2) Sauté the mushrooms in the skillet about three minutes, sprinkling with flour. Empty the broth and Marsala—bringing to a boil.
3) Allow it to simmer about five minutes to thicken.

4 Points per Serving
Yields: Four Servings
Prep Time: Zero (except to put it together) Cooking time: 20 Minutes

Mexican Chicken Breasts *

Ingredients
1 cup salsa
16 ounces skinless chicken breasts (boneless also)
1 (1 ¼-ounce) Package taco seasonings

¼ cup fat-free sour cream

Instructions
1) Heat the oven at 375°F. Prepare a casserole dish with some cooking spray.
2) Use a re-sealable plastic bag to combine the breasts and taco seasonings—shake well to coat evenly.
3) Put the chicken breasts into the dish and bake for thirty minutes.

Garnish with the salsa for the last five minutes of the cooking cycle. Add a bit of sour cream.

4 Points per Serving
Yields: Four Servings (four-ounce servings)
Prep Time: Three minutes
Cooking Time: 30 minutes

Chicken Spinach Crescent Ring *

Ingredients
5 ounces Cooked grilled chicken strips
1 Cup fresh baby spinach
4 Tablespoons reduced-fat whipped cream cheese (WW)
1 (8-ounce) can reduced-fat crescent rolls (8 rolls)
1/3 cup reduced-fat Mexican cheese (WW)

Instructions
1) Prepare a pan with some aluminum foil or use a small aluminum roasting pan. Heat the oven to 375°F.
2) Create a ring with the rolls (Points on the outer edge).
3) Spread the cream cheese, a layer of spices, spinach, and spread out the grilled chicken on the roll. Lastly, add the Mexican cheese.
4) Stretch all of the points and wrap around the mixture—tucking it under the top.
5) Bake for 14 minutes. Yummy.

3 Points per Serving
Yields: Eight Servings
Preparation Time and Cooking Times: 15 Minutes each; Total time 30 minutes

Cracking Chicken Slaw *

Ingredients
½ medium head of cabbage
1 pound ground chicken breast
12 (10-12 Ounce) Bag broccoli slaw mix
4 minced garlic cloves
1 small finely chopped onion
½ teaspoon ginger (freshly grated)
¼ cup reduced-sodium soy sauce
1 Tablespoon olive oil
Salt and pepper
One teaspoon each:
- Apple cider vinegar
- Toasted sesame oil
- Sriracha sauce

Instructions
1) Shred the cabbage.
2) Use the stovetop, and set the burner to medium heat—adding the oil to a frying pan.
3) Toss in the onions and sauté for one to two minutes. Blend in the ginger, garlic, and chicken—breaking it up with a wooden spoon—until browned.
4) Take it out of the skillet and add the broccoli, slaw, and cabbage—cooking for about four to five minutes.
5) Place the meat back in the pan and pour in the vinegar, sesame oil, Sriracha and soy sauce. Flavor with a bit more pepper and salt or Sriracha if desired.

2 Smart Points per Serving
Yields: Four Servings (1 ½ cups each)
Prep Times: Fifteen minutes
Cooking Time: Fifteen minutes

Chicken Taco Salad *

8 medium corn tortillas (cut each into 4 wedges)
4 cups romaine shredded lettuce
½ teaspoon table salt
1 Pound chicken breast (cooked and shredded)

1 cup diced tomatoes
½ cup fat-free shredded Mexican blend cheese
¼ cup salsa
½ cup fat-free sour cream
½ teaspoon adobo seasoning/ground cumin
4 sprays olive oil
½ teaspoon hot pepper sauce

Instructions
1) Coat a cookie tin/baking sheet lightly with the cooking spray.
2) Heat the oven to 400°F.
3) Lay out the tortillas on the prepared sheet—spray with some oil—add a shake of salt. Bake until a nice golden color.

4) *Build the Salad*: Begin with the lettuce, chicken, tomatoes, and lastly the cheese in four serving dishes.
5) Whisk the hot pepper sauce, salsa, sour cream, and cumin; drizzle about three tablespoons over each of the salads.

Each Serving: 7 Smart Points; 8 Points Plus; 6 points (old)
Yields: Four Servings (1 bowl per serving)
Prep time: Twenty minutes
Cook time: Ten minutes

General TSO's Chicken *

Ingredients
¾ C. chicken broth (can reduced-sodium)
2 Tbsp. sugar
2 Tbsp. Cornstarch
½ tsp. ground ginger
1 Tbsp. White wine vinegar
1 Tbsp. Low-sodium soy sauce
2 medium minced garlic cloves
2 tsp. peanut oil
2 medium chopped scallions
1 minced dried chili or ½ teaspoon red pepper flakes
2 C. cooked white rice

1 Pound chicken breasts (No skin or bones)

Instructions
1) In a medium container, whisk the sugar, broth, soy sauce, cornstarch, ginger, and vinegar; set to the side.
2) Begin by using medium-high heat and a large skillet or a wok to heat the oil. Toss in the garlic, scallions, and pepper—cook for about two minutes.
3) Combine the breasts of chicken with the scallion mixture, and continue cooking for about five minutes. Pour the sauce (from step 1) and simmer about three minutes until the sauce has thickened, and chicken is cooked.
4) Serve the tasty chicken over a bed of rice.

8 Smart Points; 8 Points Plus; 7 Points (old)
Yields: Four Servings
Preparation time is twenty minutes.
Cooking time is ten minutes.

Chicken Teriyaki & Broccoli *

Ingredients
1 Pound Uncooked chicken breasts (*skinless * boneless)
2 medium minced garlic cloves
4 medium uncooked scallions (chopped)
    Note: Use the green and white parts
2 Tablespoons teriyaki sauce
½ cup reduced sodium chicken broth
4 cups uncooked broccoli
2 cups cooked brown rice (instant/regular)

Instructions
1) Use some non-stick cooking spray to prepare a skillet using the med-high heat setting on the stovetop.
2) Cut the chicken into one-inch cubes.
3) Prepare the broccoli into florets. Place them in a microwave-safe dish in ½-inch of water. Place a cover over the bowl and cook on high for four minutes. You can also steam it in a steamer basket over a pot of water for four to five minutes.

4) Put the garlic into the pan and saute for around one minute. Put the chicken in with the garlic and let it brown about five minutes—evenly on each side.
5) Toss in the scallions—continue to cook about two minutes.
6) Pour the teriyaki sauce and broth into the mixture until the chicken is done. It should take about five minutes.
7) Add a layer (1/2 cup) of rice—chicken—and top it off with ½ cup of broccoli over the top of each of the four servings.

Points Plus Value: Seven per Serving
Yields: Four Servings
Preparation Time: 20 Min.; *Cook Time:* 13 Min.

Lemon Parmesan Chicken Piccata *

Ingredients
Pepper
Salt
1 cup chicken broth (fat-free)
2 teaspoons olive oil
¼ cup whole wheat flour
1 Tablespoon butter
4 garlic cloves
1 teaspoon cornstarch
2 Tablespoons capers
½ cup Parmesan cheese (freshly grated)
1 pound Chicken Breasts (boneless – skinless)

Instructions
1) Mince the garlic cloves. Slice the chicken into four thin fillets. Blend the pepper, salt, and flour; dredge the fillets through it shaking off any excess flour and set it aside.
2) Use the med-high heat setting, and place a large skillet on the stovetop burner. Cook the chicken about two to four minutes on each side. Take it out of the pan and set to the side.
3) *Make the Sauce*: Toss in the garlic and saute for one minute. Lower the heat to medium-low—empty the milk

and broth to the mixture; bring to a boiling. Flavor with the pepper and salt.

4) Blend in the capers and Parmesan cheese—letting it simmer for around two minutes to thicken. Add one tablespoon of water with the cornstarch, and blend the mixture into the pan.

5) Pour in the lemon juice and place the chicken back into the pan to warm up for a couple of minutes.

Smart Points Per Serving: Six
Yields: Four Servings
Prep Time: Preparation time is ten minutes. Cooking time is fifteen minutes.

Pork

Baked Pork Cutlets

Ingredients
½ cup dry whole wheat breadcrumbs
1 Pound trimmed pork tenderloin
1 teaspoon sugar
½ teaspoon each:

- Salt
- Onion powder
- Sugar
- Paprika

4 teaspoons cornstarch
1 large (lightly beaten) egg white
4 teaspoons canola oil

Instructions
1) Use some cooking spray to prepare a baking sheet (with a rim).
2) Heat the oven to 400°F.
3) Slice the tenderloin at a 45° angle into four long – thin fillets.
4) Combine the salt, paprika, onion powder, breadcrumbs, and sugar in a shallow dish.
5) Drizzle with the oil while mashing with a fork to blend. Gently whip the egg white in a separate container. Add

some of the cornstarch to coat the slices of pork—patting evenly on each side.
6) Dredge the pork through the egg, and then breading mixture. (Throw the leftover mix away.)
7) Put the pork in the oven and bake about fourteen to sixteen minutes or until the internal temperature reaches 145°F.

Plus+ 5 Points per Serving
Yields: Four Servings
Cooking Time: Fourteen to Sixteen minutes

Pork Barbecue Sandwiches with Coleslaw *

Ingredients
1 Pound lean pork tenderloin
3 tablespoons mayonnaise (reduced-calorie)
3 1/3 Tablespoons BBQ sauce (3 T. plus 1 t.)
1 teaspoon apple cider vinegar
1/8 teaspoon black pepper
1 Tablespoon water
3 tablespoons sliced scallions
2 cups coleslaw mix (Carrots and cabbage shredded)
4 mixed-grain burger buns

Instructions
1) Prepare a roasting pan with cooking spray or aluminum foil.
2) Heat the oven to 450°F.
3) Put the pork in the baking pan and coat it with two tablespoons of the barbecue sauce. Bake it for about 25 minutes or to 160F on the meat thermometer.
4) Let the pork rest or sit for ten minutes.
5) In the meantime, whip the pepper, vinegar, water, and mayonnaise in a mixing dish until creamy smooth. Blend in the scallions and coleslaw mix—tossing to coat evenly.
6) Slice the roast into about twenty slices—placing five slices on the bottom half of each roll. Drizzle with some sauce and top with a serving of ½ cup of the slaw. Top it with the top half of the bun.

Yields: Four Servings (1 sandwich)
Six Points per serving
Preparation Time: Ten minutes
Cooking Time: Twenty-five minutes

Seafood and Fish

These are just several delightful fish and seafood and fish recipes you will simply adore!

Crab Cake Burgers *

Ingredients
1 Lb. Crabmeat
½ C. panko breadcrumbs
1 lightly beaten egg
4 dashes hot sauce
¼ C. light mayonnaise
¼ teaspoon freshly ground pepper
One teaspoon each:
• Onion powder
• Celery seed
¼ teaspoon black pepper
2 tablespoons minced chives
1 Tablespoon each:
• Lemon juice
• Dijon mustard
2 teaspoons butter (unsalted)
1 tablespoon of Olive oil

Optional:
• Favorite Toppings
• Whole wheat buns

Instructions
1) Combine the breadcrumbs, crab, mayonnaise, egg, mustard, chives, celery seed, lemon juice, onion powder, hot sauce, and pepper in a large mixing container.
2) Shape the mixture into six patties.

3) On the stovetop, select the medium heat setting and pour the butter and oil into a nonstick skillet.
4) Wait until the butter quits foaming and add the patties cooking approximately four minutes on each side.

You can serve on the buns, but the points are not added for the bun.

*4 Points (+) Per Serving (*Not counting the buns*)*
Yields: Six Servings

Crab Quesadillas *

Ingredients
¼ cup chopped tomato
8 ounces imitation crabmeat
1 Can diced green chilies (4-ounce)
2 Tablespoons chopped green bell pepper
½ cup shredded Cheddar or Monterey Jack cheese
4 (eight-inch) tortillas

1) *Instructions*
2) Set the oven the 425°F.
3) Combine the bell peppers, tomatoes, chilies, crabmeat, and cheese.
4) Use some cooking spray on one side of the tortilla—flip it over—spoon ¼ of the mixture onto the unsprayed side and fold in half.
5) After all four are prepared, put them –uncovered—on a baking tin and bake for ten minutes.

Yields: Four Servings (1 sandwich)
9 Smart Points; 8 Points Plus; 6 Points (old)
Prep Time: Five minutes
Cooking Time: Fifteen minutes

Grilled Pineapple Halibut *

Ingredients
4 (6-ounce) 1 ¼ Pounds - halibut fillets
2 cups (½ medium) pineapple
1 Tablespoon lime zest

1 teaspoon table salt
¼ teaspoon cayenne pepper
2 Tablespoons Each:
- Lime juice
- Divided - unpacked - light brown sugar
- Fresh Ginger root (divided)

Non-fat Cooking spray

Instructions
1) Preheat and spray the grill with the cooking spray.
2) Cut the halibut into ½-inch steaks. Slice the pineapple lengthwise into ½-inch spears.
3) In a re-sealable plastic bag, pour in the lime juice, zest, salt, the cayenne pepper, and one tablespoon each of the ginger and brown sugar—shake and combine.
4) Put the fish into the bag and seal, shake and allow it to marinate for twenty minutes—flipping once.
5) In a second plastic bag, add the remainder of the brown sugar, pineapple, and ginger—seal and marinate for five minutes. Take the pineapple out and pour the rest of the juices into the 'fish' bag.
6) Grill the pineapple for about eight minutes—flipping once.
7) Put the pineapple on a platter and cover with some aluminum foil.
8) Using direct heat on the grill; brush the fish with the marinade and grill for three to four minutes per side.
9) Add to the serving platter with the pineapple and enjoy.

Smart Points Per Serving: Four
Yields: Serving Size: 1 fillet + ½ cup of pineapple (Four Servings)

Lime-Honey Salmon *

Ingredients
1 Pound Salmon
1 Tablespoon olive oil
¼ cup fresh parsley
Juice of 2 limes
1 Tablespoon honey

4 minced garlic cloves
1 teaspoon each:
- Salt
- Ground cumin

Instructions
1) Slice the salmon into four fillets. Finely chop the parsley and mince the garlic cloves.
2) Use some cooking spray or parchment paper to line a baking sheet. Heat the oven to 400°F.
3) Blend all of the listed items in a small mixing container.
4) Put the salmon on the baking sheet and brush it with the sauce. Coat each one evenly.
5) Roast the salmon for about ten to twelve minutes.

Enjoy with a garnish of lime slices.

5 Smart Points per Serving
Yields: Four Servings (1 fillet per serving)
Preparation Time: Five Minutes; *Cooking Time*: Ten Minutes

Maple Glazed Salmon *

Ingredients
4 (6-ounce) skinless wild salmon fillets
3 Tbsp. Reduced-Sodium soy sauce
3 Tbsp. Pure maple syrup
1 smashed garlic clove
1 Tbsp. Sriracha hot sauce

Instructions
1) Mix the Sriracha, garlic, soy sauce, and maple syrup in a dish and pour into a plastic large Ziploc bag with the salmon.
2) Marinate the mixture for 20 to 60 minutes. Turn it occasionally.
3) Grease a baking pan with some cooking spray. Heat the oven to 425°F.
4) Pat the fish dry and empty the marinade into a small pan.
5) Put the fish on the baking pan and bake for eight to ten minutes.

6) In the meantime, using medium heat, simmer the marinade into a glaze and spoon before you serve your delicious salmon.

7 Smart Points per Serving
Yields: Four Servings (1 piece per serving)
Cooking Time: 10 Minutes

Baked Parmesan Fish

Ingredients
4-ounces (one-inch thickness) frozen salmon/favorite fish fillet
1 tsp. Worcestershire Sauce for chicken
1 Tbsp. Sliced green onion/fresh chives
¼ C. salad dressing/light mayonnaise
2 T. grated parmesan cheese

Directions
1) Heat the oven temperature to 450°F. Prepare a baking dish with a small amount of oil or cooking spray.
2) Be sure the fish are thawed. Pat each piece dry with paper towels and set them to the side.
3) Combine everything (for the sauce) except for the fish in a mixing container. Spread the mixture over your fish of choice and bake for 8 to 12 minutes.

Yields: Four Servings
Points Plus+ 4 per Serving
Cooking time: Eight to Twelve Minutes

Broiled Scallops

Ingredients
Pepper and Salt to taste
12 sea scallops
2 Tbsp. Fresh parsley (chopped)
2 Tbsp. Olive oil
1 Tbsp. Lemon juice
Serving: Lemon Wedges

Instructions

1) Heat the broiler on the high setting.
2) Place the scallops in some towels to dry.
3) Flavor the scallops with the pepper and salt.
4) Place the scallops on a baking sheet.
5) Thoroughly clean the countertops.
6) Mix the lemon juice and olive oil; brush on the scallops lightly.
7) Broil for five to six minutes—flip them—continue cooking for another five to six more minutes.
8) Garnish with a squeeze of lemon and some chopped parsley.

Smart Points: 6 per Serving
Yields: Four Servings (four-ounce servings)
Prep Time is ten minutes.
Cooking Time is twelve minutes.

Shrimp with a Spicy Sauce *

Ingredients
1 Lb. shrimp (uncooked)
1 T. (divided) olive oil
4 teaspoons minced garlic (divided)
¾ teaspoon salt (divided)
½ teaspoon crushed red pepper flakes
½ cup fresh chopped basil
1 (28-ounce) can tomatoes with juices

Instructions
1) Coarsely crush the tomatoes. Peel and devein the shrimp.
2) Using the stovetop; place a skillet and add one teaspoon of the oil along with one teaspoon of the garlic, shrimp, and ¼ teaspoon of salt. Sauté for about two to three minutes. Place onto a dish.
3) In the same skillet; add another teaspoon of the oil using low heat—toss in the remainder of the garlic and red pepper. Sauté until the aroma takes your senses—about thirty seconds.
4) Add the rest of the salt and tomatoes to the skillet— simmering using the med-low setting.

5) Be sure to scrape the flavorful morsels stuck to the bottom of the skillet. Continue cooking about ten minutes.
6) Return the juices and shrimp to the mixture, and completely heat. Blend in the basil until it wilts.
7) Take the skillet off the burner and add the remainder of the oil—flavoring with the red pepper.

Note: Use about 21 to 25 shrimp for each pound. Choose the large-sized ones.
Prep Time is 13 minutes and the *cooking time* is also 13 minutes.
Yields: Four Servings
Two Points per Serving

Shrimp Scampi *

Ingredients
1 ¼ Pounds medium shrimp
4 tsp. olive oil
6 – 8 minced garlic cloves
½ C. each:
- Low-sodium chicken broth
- Dry white wine

¼ C. (+) 1 Tbsp. minced parsley
¼ C. fresh squeezed lemon juice
¼ tsp. each:
- Black pepper
- Salt

4 lemon slices.

Instructions
1) Peel the shrimp leaving the tails on and remove the veins.
2) Heat the oil in a large pan and sauté the shrimp two to three minutes, until just showing pink. Blend in the garlic and sauté for about thirty more seconds. Use a slotted spoon to place the shrimp on a warming platter.
3) Add the wine, broth, ¼ cup of the pepper, salt, parsley, and lemon juice in the skillet—bringing it to a boil. Continue cooking until the sauce is lowered in half by volume.

4) Empty the sauce over the tops of the shrimp and garnish using the remainder of the parsley and a couple of lemon slices.

Plus+ 4 per Serving
Yields: Four Servings

Tilapia Parmesan *

Ingredients
2 Pounds Tilapia fillets
¼ C. softened butter
½ C. Parmesan cheese
3 Tbsp. Mayonnaise
¼ tsp. each:
- Black pepper
- Dried basil

2 Tbsp. Lemon juice
1/8 tsp. each:
- Celery salt
- Onion powder

Instructions
1) Cover a baking sheet with some aluminum foil and set it to the side.
2) Heat the oven to the broil function.
3) Blend all of the listed ingredients in a container and mix well.
4) Broil the tilapia for two to three minutes in the prepared pan.
5) Turn the fillets over and continue grilling for about two to three additional minutes.
6) Use the parmesan mixture and cover the fillets—returning them to the broiler until lightly browned—around two more minutes.

Six Points per Serving
Yields: Eight Servings
Preparation time: five minutes; Cook time: nine minutes

Baked Tuna Melt *

Ingredients
1 Can (6-ounce) Tuna
½ cup processed American cheese
2 chopped – medium celery stalks
¼ cup light mayonnaise
1/8 tsp. Salt
¼ tsp. pepper
1 Tbsp. Instant minced onion
12 Slices whole wheat bread

Instructions
Set the oven to 350°F.
1) Drain and break the tuna apart.
2) Dice the cheese. Wash and chop the celery.
3) Mix the remainder of the ingredients in a medium mixing container.
4) Prepare the sandwiches and place each one – individually—in foil and bake for 20 minutes until piping hot.
5) Cool slightly and enjoy!

8 Smart Points/6 Points Plus - per serving
Yields: Six Sandwiches
Prep Time: Five minutes; *Cooking Time*: Twenty minutes

Salads

Layered BLT Salad

Ingredients
4 C. lettuce (finely shredded)
¼ cup bacon bits
1/3 C. shredded Cheddar cheese (reduced-fat)
1 ½ C. chopped fresh tomatoes
4 slices toasted and cubed (reduced-calorie white bread)
½ C. Thousand Island dressing (fat-free)
1 tsp. dried parsley flakes
¼ C. fat-free mayonnaise

Instructions
1) Layer the lettuce and tomatoes along with the toast cubes, bacon bits, and Cheddar cheese in a large salad bowl.
2) In a separate dish, mix the parsley flakes, mayonnaise, and Thousand Island dressing.
3) Spread the dressing over the salad, cover, and put in the fridge for about thirty minutes.

Plus+ 4 per Serving
Yields: Four servings

Tuna Salad & Stuffed Tomatoes *

Ingredients
1 (20-ounce) Can Tuna in Water
¼ Cup Each:
- Fat-free mayonnaise
- Non-fat Green Yogurt (plain)

3 Stalks chopped celery
1 chopped hard-boiled egg
½ small diced red onions
1 - Tbsp. each:
- Dijon mustard
- Sweet pickle relish

2 Tbsp. Minced fresh parsley
Pepper and salt if desired
6 Large tomatoes

Instructions
1) Drain the can of tuna, and rinse thoroughly. Drain again.
2) Combine everything in a large container, but OMIT the tomatoes.
3) Cut off the tops of each tomato and de-seed them forming a dish/bowl.
4) Fill them with the tune and serve right away.

Points + for each Serving: Value 4
Yields: (1/2 Cup tuna salad + 1 tomato) Six Servings
Prep: 15 minutes; Cook time: Zero

Sides

Angel Hair Pasta & Eggplant *

Ingredients
1 medium sweet red pepper
1 medium uncooked eggplant (baby-variety)
¾ teaspoon table salt (divided)
2 large fresh tomatoes
1 spray of olive oil cooking spray
1 medium minced clove garlic
¼ teaspoon crushed red pepper flakes
1/8 teaspoon black pepper
1 (8-ounce) package uncooked angel hair pasta
½ cup reduced-sodium vegetable broth
2 Tablespoons each Fresh Minced:
- Chives
- Basil

4 ounces crumbled feta cheese

Instructions
1) Cut the red pepper into 8-inch strips and the eggplant into 1/3 to ½-inch thick rounds. Coarsely chop the tomatoes.
2) Prepare the pasta according to its labeling instructions.
3) Coat the veggies with the cooking spray and ½ teaspoon of salt.
4) Set the grill on the medium setting—placing the pepper and eggplant into the basket—or on a piece of foil with holes poked in to let the smoke seep into them.
5) Cook for approximately two to three minutes on each side. Take them from the grill and cool—cut into bite-sized pieces and set to the side.
6) Prepare a skillet over low-medium heat using the cooking spray. Toss in the garlic and sauté for one minute—blend in the tomatoes and continue sautéing for one more minute.
7) Stir in the remainder of the veggies and ingredients (except for the cheese) and continue cooking for approximately two to three minutes.

8) Pour in the pasta and toss. Blend in the cheese when ready to eat.

Notes: You can also roast the veggies in the oven at 425°F. You can substitute yellow squash, sliced zucchini or red onion for the eggplant if you want a change of menu.

Smart Points per Serving: 6
Yields: Serves Six
Prep Time: Sixteen minutes; *Cook Time*: Twelve minutes

Ham and Noodle Casserole

Ingredients
4 ounces No Yolks noodle substitute
8 ounces turkey ham
1 Can (10 ¾-ounces) low-fat cream of mushroom soup
½ cup each:
- Chopped onions
- Fat-free milk
2 ounces white cheddar cheese (shredded)

Instructions
1) Cook and cube the ham. Prepare the noodles and drain.
2) Heat the oven to 375°F.
3) Use some cooking spray to grease an eight-inch square dish/pan, and set to the side.
4) Combine the onions, ham, and noodles—mixing well—set aside.
5) Prepare the milk and soup—mix—and pour over the ham mixture, stirring in until combined.
6) Add it to the dish, sprinkle with cheese, and heat until thoroughly heated—usually about twenty minutes.

Plus+ 5 per Serving
Yields: Eight Servings
Cook time: 10 minutes

Spaghetti Carbonara

Ingredients
3 slices reduced fat bacon (one-inch cubes
1 (8-ounces) Package of whole wheat spaghetti
1large egg white (+) 1 large egg (beaten)
1 minced garlic clove

Instructions
1) Pour a little salt into a pot of boiling water. Add the spaghetti and cook as required by the panel of instructions. Drain—but reserve ½ cup of the water—set to the side.
2) Cook the bacon over medium heat in a large skillet for approximately four to six minutes. Blend in the garlic—alone for thirty seconds—and add the spaghetti. Toss to coat well and take off of the burner.
3) Add the Parmesan and eggs, whisking until the eggs are a bit thicker (not scrambled). You don/t want the sauce to be thick; but if it is, add a little of the reserved pasta water until you have it the right consistency for your taste.
4) Top with the bits of bacon.

6 Smart Points; 6 Points Plus per Serving
Yields: Five Servings
Preparation time is ten minutes.
Cooking time is twenty-five minutes.

Tuscan Pasta *

Ingredients
1 Can diced tomatoes (28-ounce)
1 Can tomato sauce (8-ounce)
½ tsp. ground black pepper
2 tsp. Garlic powder
2 tsp. Italian seasoning
2 T. Olive oil
½ tsp. salt
1 small chopped onion
1 (8-ounce) Package sliced mushrooms

1 Pound sliced yellow squash/zucchini
6 ounces Pasta (linguine or spaghetti)
Optional: Sugar and Shredded Parmesan cheese

Instructions
1) Don't drain the tomatoes.
2) Combine the seasonings, sugar, tomatoes, and sauce in a pan; bring it to a boil using medium heat.
3) Reduce the temperature setting and simmer twenty minutes, covered.
4) Heat a skillet using the med-high setting and add the oil. Toss in the mushrooms, onions, and zucchini—continuing to simmer for about four more minutes.
5) Blend the veggies into the tomato sauce.
6) In the meantime, prepare the pasta (according to manufacturer's instructions), and drain.
7) Put the pasta in the serving dish and blend the veggie mixture; toss and add a sprinkle of the Parmesan cheese.

Yields: Six Servings
Plus+ 5 per Serving

Baked Ziti

Ingredients
8 ounces each:
- Uncooked ziti pasta
- Hot or mild salsa
- Regular/salt-free tomato sauce

¾ cup fat-free ricotta cheese
1 (11-ounce) Can drained corn
1 cup fat-free mozzarella cheese
1 teaspoon dried oregano
4 ounces drained & chopped green chili peppers
2 tablespoons fat-free grated parmesan cheese
1/8 teaspoon pepper

Instructions
1) Heat the oven in advance to 375°F. Use a cooking spray to oil an eight-inch baking dish/pan.

2) Prepare the ziti noodles according to the package directions using the lowest amount of time. Drain.
3) Combine the salsa and tomato sauce in a small container.
4) Combine half of the mozzarella and half of ricotta in a big bowl. Pour in ½ of the sauce, with the oregano, chilies, pepper, and corn. Add the ziti (cooked), and mix.
5) Scoop the creation into the baking dish—adding the sauce on top—sprinkling with the rest of the two kinds of cheese.
6) Place a lid or some aluminum foil over the meal, and bake for twenty minutes—uncover and continue baking about ten to fifteen more minutes.

Points: Plus+ 7 per Serving
Yields: One cup per serving

Pizza Pasta Salad

Ingredients
1 ½ cups uncooked Rotelle pasta (spoke wheels)
1 (8-ounce) block Mozzarella cheese
½ cup sliced green onions
2 Cups halved cherry tomatoes
½ cup diced green bell pepper
10 slices pepperoni (quartered)
½ Cup light Italian dressing
¼ teaspoon Italian seasoning
Pinch of black pepper

Instructions
1) Cut the cheese into ½-inch cubes.
2) Prepare the pasta according to the package instructions. Use cold water to rinse the Rotelle and drain.
3) In a big container, mix each of the ingredients along with the pasta—tossing well.
4) Place a cover over the contents and refrigerate for about two to three hours before it is mealtime.

6 Smart Points per Serving
Yields: 9 (1/2 cup Servings)

Sautéed Spinach and Garlic *

Ingredients
32 ounces fresh spinach (baby leaves)
4 garlic cloves (thinly sliced)
1 Tbsp. Olive oil
¼ tsp. Red pepper flakes
½ tsp. Table salt

Directions
1) Using medium heat on the stovetop; add and heat the oil in a frying pan. Toss the garlic and cook to a sizzle approximately 2 ½ minutes. Take it out of the pan using a slotted spoon.
2) Add about half of the spinach into the skillet tossing for about 1 ½- to 2 minutes or until the spinach wilts and place in a small container.
3) Add the remainder of the spinach to the pan (throw away the residual liquid), cooking it for 1 ½- to two minutes also. Take it off of the burner.
4) Sprinkle with the pepper flakes and salt for extra flavor—tossing to coat the greens evenly.

2 Points plus Value per Serving
Yields: Six Servings (2/3 cup servings)
Prep Times: 8 minutes: *Cook Time*: 7 minutes

Veggies

Sautéed Tomatoes and Cauliflower *

Ingredients
8 cups uncooked fresh cauliflower florets
4 teaspoons (divided) extra-virgin oil
¼ cup of water
1 Tablespoon garlic (minced)
2 cups halved grape tomatoes
½ teaspoon black pepper
¾ teaspoon kosher salt

Instructions
1) Use the stovetop and place a twelve-inch skillet on a med-high burner. Warm up two teaspoons of the oil and toss in the cauliflower. Cover the skillet—stirring occasionally. If needed you can add a few tablespoons of water. It should be ready between six to eight minutes.
2) Blend in the garlic, tomatoes, pepper, salt, and remainder of the oil. Stir about three minutes until the tomatoes and cauliflower are tender.

Option: You can also roast this for a change of pace!

Points + per Serving: Value 2
Yields: Six Servings (one-cup each)
Prep: 10 minutes; *Cook Time:* 12 minutes

Cheesy Cauliflower Bake *

Ingredients
4 C. small cauliflower florets
¾ cup shredded 2% sharp Cheddar cheese
3 ounces Velveeta 2% (1/2-inch cubes)
¼ cup sliced almonds
¼ teaspoon ground nutmeg
1 cup corn flakes

Instructions
1) Heat the oven in advance at 375°F.
2) Place the cauliflower in an ovenproof 8 x 9-inch square dish. Cook on high for three to four minutes.
3) Garnish with the remainder of ingredients and bake in the prepared oven until browned, usually for 12 to 14 minutes.

Plus+ 4 per Serving
Yields: Six (½ cup Servings)

Zucchini Carpaccio

Ingredients
½ of a lemon
2 medium zucchini ends
4 teaspoons olive oil
1 cup baby arugula

Fresh black pepper
Kosher salt to taste

Instructions
1) Cut off and slice the ends (1/16) of the zucchini with a
   <u>mandolin</u>.
2) Blend the juice and oil.
3) Place one layer of zucchini over the base of the serving
   platter. Flavor with some pepper and salt and a drizzle of
   the oil/juice—continue layering until all ingredients are
   used up—let marinade for a minimum of ten minutes.
4) Garnish with the fresh arugula and shaved Parmesan.
Yields: Four Servings
2 Smart Points
Total Preparation and Cooking times are 20 minutes.

Conclusion

Thank for making it through to the end of *Weight Watchers: Quick and Easy Recipes for Fast Weight Loss.* Let's hope it was informative and provided you with all of the tools you need to achieve your goals, whether the reasons are for weight loss or other reasons.

The next step is to discover which delicious recipe to tempt your taste buds with whether it is for breakfast, lunch, dinner, or snacks. You have the answers now.

As a reminder, here are a few of them as a reminder of some of the tasty foods you can enjoy and remain within the limits of your Weight Watchers Plan:

- **Ham and Noodle Casserole** *

- **Good Morning Wrap** *

- **Chicken Noodle Soup (WW Style)** *

- **Quinoa Black Bean Salad** *

- **Dutch Babies (Pancake Type)** *

- **Chicken Taco Salad** *

- **Filet Mignon & Caramelized Onions**

- **Kiwi & Banana Salad***

- **Baked Ziti***

- **Baked Parmesan Fish**

Finally, if you found this book useful in any way, a review on Amazon is always appreciated!

Description

If you're the kinda person that " hasn't got time to eat healthy" then this is the book for you! We have carefully selected and explained each and every meal for you.

Through our meal plan you should expect to lose weight over the 30 day period! With little to no effort. Our diet is designed to be as easy and care free while still letting you enjoy your life and not starve yourself to death!

We also go to the lengths of teaching you how to understand the process of losing weight and what you should eat and at what times!

Go ahead an download your personal copy of this treasure; you will want to keep close by in your library of recipes. You can stay prepared with your meal plans when you have the time to look ahead during a short break from work or other activities.

Don't waste any more time worrying about weight lose purchase this book today; you will be glad you have your personal copy of *healthy Eating: 30 Days of Clean Eating; The Perfect Cookbook To Start A Healthy Diet And Still Enjoy Some Sneaky Sweets* any time you need to have it as a reference.